The Smoothies for Runners Book

36 Delicious Super Smoothie Recipes Designed to Support the Specific Needs Runners and Joggers (Achieve Your Optimum Health, Performance, Endurance and Physique Goals)

Lars Andersen

Published by Nordic Standard Publishing

Atlanta, Georgia USA

NORDICSTANDARD PUBLISHING

ISBN 978-1-484144-96-1

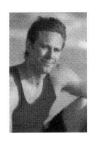

Lars Andersen

What Our Readers Are Saying

"When I wake up for my pre-work run, I don't have much time to spare - these recipes are ideal and tasty too. Perfect."

★★★★☆ **Kris Chapman (Melissa, TX)**

"I'm always looking forward to the next smoothie... I'm seriously considering taking all my meals in smoothie format"

★★★★★ **Rachel Pruitt (Harrisburg, PA)**

"The 'healthy' products in my local supermarket taste nowhere near as good as these do (not to mention they cost 5x as much as making my own)"

★★★★★ **Jon Robinson (Onego, WV)**

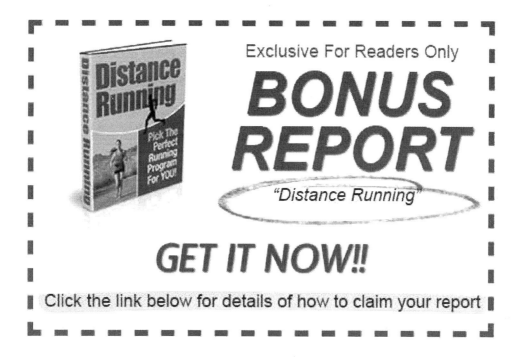

Exclusive Bonus Download: Distance Running

Discover How You Can Increase Your Running In A Matter Of A Few Months!

Now, you can implement the same kind of training that runners use to train for marathons, races and other running events! You can steal the strategies that runners use to get to the next level. You will be able to discover the secrets that they use to get to where they are at today.

If your running speed is not up to par, this report, " Distance Running - Pick The Perfect Running Program For YOU! " , can help you get up to speed on the level that you need to be at with your running. There are six different running programs that explain how you can do just that, along with other tips that are crucial to your running success. This could be the most important thing that you will ever read to make those strides that you need to make in your running pursuits. This report will explain how you can train to be like some of the other runners that are involved in different races and marathons. Before you know it, you will be running in some of the most well-known running events and being able to win, just because of the training that you received.

You will learn about the training involved:

- One of the first thing that you have to do every day while you're training
- How to keep your back and hamstrings strong

- What kind of training to incorporate on the weekends
- The average distance that you should train
- Why you should have a schedule
- How many days a week runners train
- What you should incorporate in your training
- What you should do in between training and running
- And Much Much More!

Go to the end of this book for the download link for this Bonus

---

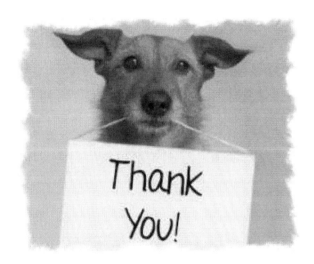

Thank you for downloading my book. Please REVIEW this book on Amazon. I need your feedback to make the next edition better. Thank you so much!

Books by This Author

The Smoothies for Runners Book

Juices for Runners

Smoothies for Cyclists

Juices for Cyclists

Paleo Diet for Cyclists

Smoothies for Triathletes

Juices for Triathletes

Paleo Diet for Triathletes

Smoothies for Strength

Juices for Strength

Paleo Diet for Strength

Paleo Diet Smoothies for Strength

Smoothies for Golfers

Juices for Golfers

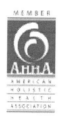

Table of Contents

HOW TO USE THIS BOOK 8

INTRODUCTION 8

SUPPLEMENTS 9

GET CREATIVE - HOW TO CREATE YOUR OWN SMOOTHIE 10

SUGAR COMES IN MANY FORMS 10

CARBOHYDRATE SMOOTHIES 11

    COFFEE DELIGHT SMOOTHIE (POST-RUN) 12

    BANANA DELIGHT (PRE-RUN) 13

    DATES BOOST (PRE-RUN) 14

    COCOA SMOOTHIE (PRE-RUN) 15

    FRISKY SMOOTHIE (POST-RUN) 16

    BANANA DELIGHT SMOOTHIE (POST-RUN) 17

    FRUITILICIOUS SMOOTHIE (POST-RUN) 18

    CHOCOLATE SMOOTHIE (POST-RUN) 19

    CHOCÓ- COFFEE SMOOTHIE (PRE-RUN) 20

    MANGO SMOOTHIE (POST-RUN) 21

    FRUITY PUNCH (POST-RUN) 22

    BUTTER MILK SMOOTHIES (PRE-RUN) 23

    OATS SMOOTHIE (PRE-RUN) 24

    PINEAPPLE COCONUT SMOOTHIE (POST-RUN) 25

    POWER- PACKED SMOOTHIE (POST-RUN) 26

MULTIVITAMIN SMOOTHIES 28

    BLUEBERRY-AVOCADO PUNCH (PRE-RUN) 29

    VEGETABLE SMOOTHIE (POST-RUN) 30

    SMOOTHIES RICH IN VITAMIN C (POST-RUN) 31

    CHERRIES SMOOTHIE (PRE-RUN) 32

    REHYDRATING SMOOTHIES (POST-RUN) 33

    VITAMIN A RICH SMOOTHIE (PRE-RUN) 34

    CARROT SMOOTHIE (PRE-RUN) 35

    CARROT TOMATO DELIGHT (POST-RUN) 36

    KIWI COOLER (PRE-RUN) 37

    PROTEIN RICH SMOOTHIES 38

    CHOCOLATE SMOOTHIE WITH PEANUT BUTTER (PRE-RUN) 39

    BANANA WITH PEANUT BUTTER SMOOTHIE (PRE-RUN) 40

    PROTEIN SMOOTHIE (POST-RUN) 41

    TOFU CHERRY SMOOTHIE (POST-RUN) 42

    TOFU STRAWBERRY SMOOTHIE (POST-RUN) 43

Eggs And Nutmeg Smoothie (Post-Run)...44

Protein Rich Pumpkin Smoothie (Post-Run)..45

GREEN SMOOTHIES...**46**

Pineapple Spinach Smoothie (Pre-Run)..47

Vitamins Rich Smoothie (Post-Run) 48

Cooler Smoothie (Pre-Run)..49

Spinach with Oats Smoothie (Pre-Run)..50

Refresher Smoothie (Pre-Run)...51

EXCLUSIVE BONUS DOWNLOAD: DISTANCE RUNNING...**52**

ONE LAST THING......**54**

Disclaimer

How to Use this Book

As I convenient feature, I've categorized each recipe in different sections in the clickable Table of Content for you to quickly navigate to them when you're preparing these smoothies. They are categorized in either Carbohydrate Rich Smoothies, Multivitamin Rich Smoothies, Protein Rich Smoothies, or Green Smoothies. Also each recipe will have an additional category for recommended consumption, either for (Pre-Run) or (Post-Run).

Introduction

As the days become warmer, you may begin feeling the effects of thirst, getting in shape for upcoming races, and of course, beach season!

Here's the solution: Smoothies. These bright, fruity concoctions refresh your taste buds and provide vital nutrients for fitness and health. You can fix a smoothie as an uplifting afternoon treat, breakfast substitute, or post-workout reward. These beverages often contain more natural nutrients than energy drinks and juices.

Fruits in smoothies contain antioxidants and fiber that will improve your immune system and help your muscles recover more rapidly from a taxing workout. Their phytochemicals help defend you against diabetes, high blood pressure and certain cancers.

Include bananas in your smoothie, which give you complex carbs that can be converted to energy. Mangos help your muscles to function with Vitamin C and potassium, and they replace lost electrolytes. Pineapple packs a punch with a vitamin called bromelain that helps reduce inflammation from training.

Supplements

Depending on your needs, there are various supplements you can add to any of the smoothies in this book. Here are some of the most common mix-in proteins and nutrients:

Omega 3 fatty acids

If you aren't into fish, smoothies that contain omega 3 fatty acids in the form of flax may be your best option. Omega 3 fatty acids reduce high levels of triglycerides, which can lead to heart disease.

Monounsaturated Fats

You're unlikely to choose an added ingredient with the word "fat" in it, so just know that on the menu monounsaturated fats are in nuts. They reduce your LDLs (the bad cholesterol) without lowering your HDL (the good cholesterol). Almonds are especially heart-healthy and provide minerals that will help you to build muscle.

Soy Protein

Soy products can help you lower your LDL cholesterol levels.

Cocoa Powder

Heart-healthy, sugar free, and tastes like chocolate!

Stevia

Often used as a substitute for sugar, this natural sweetener contains no calories or carbohydrates.

L-Carnitine

This vitamin can improves heart health. It can also improve your regulation of insulin or glucose and suppress your appetite.

Other common supplements include green tea, which provides you with energy; agave, a sweetener with a low glycemic index, and ginger, for more antioxidants. Protein powder is also frequently used and will help you build muscle.

Get Creative - How to Create Your Own Smoothie

Once you have tried all the combinations in this book and have an idea of which flavors you like best, why not experiment with creating your own smoothies – it's great fun!

- Gather some fresh or frozen fruit in a blender. Strawberries, bananas, kiwis, and oranges are favorite fruits, but don't forget about blueberries, raspberries and others that are high in antioxidants! Avoid frozen fruit that comes in preservative-rich syrup.
- If the recipe calls for it, pour in milk – you can use skim, almond or soy milk for lower calorie content.
- A dash of orange juice or lemonade will add a burst of citrus zest. Cocoa powder also adds that chocolaty taste without any added sugar.
- Toss in some veggies, such as spinach, if you don't mind the green color. They won't affect the taste much, and you'll be adding more of those replenishing-antioxidants.
- Place it in the fridge, or add ice cubes to quickly chill your beverage.
- Pour, toast to your health, and enjoy! Your body will be in shape for the big race before you know it.

Sugar Comes in Many forms

Obviously if a smoothie contains peanut butter or chocolate, you know it's probably going to be high in sugar. What you may not realize is that fruit juices tend to be very high in sugar too and so are best consumed in post-run smoothies only.

Carbohydrate Smoothies

Carbohydrates are an important source of energy for the body. They are easily digested and do not produce gastric stress. Studies have proved that a diet rich in Carbohydrates helps to support those following exercise regimes whilst improving performance too. The Glycemic Index is a system through which foods are measured and listed in order, as per the rate at which they release energy into the bloodstream. Carbohydrates are divided by their Glycemic Index number into two main categories:

High Glycemic Index (high GI)

Foods which are high GI are easily absorbed by the body and hence can be used for Post Run Smoothies. Smoothies rich in sugar content and which contain more glucose are high GI carbohydrate smoothies. The High GI carbohydrates can be mixed with low GI and effectively made into a smoothie that replenishes energy levels after a workout or a run.

Low Glycemic Index (Low GI)

Foods which are absorbed slowly by the body and give out energy slowly are said to be 'Low GI'. These are used as Pre Run smoothies and contain oats, vegetables and pulses. The low GI carbohydrate containing smoothies provide energy for longer times and hence are useful to drink before workout or running. The Low GI carbohydrates help to keep the glycogen rates high provide steady energy to the body.

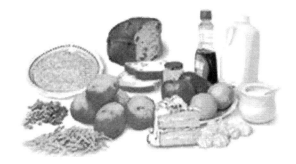

Coffee Delight Smoothie (Post-Run)

The caffeine in this smoothie helps in the recovery of athletes. The Journal of Applied Physiology states that a combination of caffeine with carbohydrates is a far better remedy for restoring glycogen in muscles as compared to the carbohydrates alone. So enjoy these for a speedy recovery!

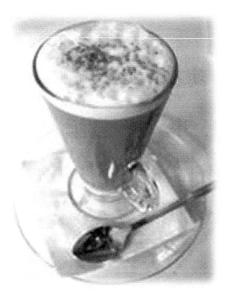

Preparation time	10 minutes
Ready time	10 minutes
Calories	157 Cal
Total Fat	5.6 g
Cholesterol	10 mg
Sodium	53 mg
Total Carbohydrates	22.6 g
Dietary fibers	2.3 g
Sugars	15.7 g
Protein	6.1 g
Vitamin C	0.09
Vitamin A	0.05
Iron	0.02
Calcium	0.16

Ingredients

- 1 banana
- 1 cup coffee
- 1 cup milk(fat-free)
- 10 crushed almonds
- 1 teaspoon sugar

Method

- Mix all the ingredients except the almonds in a blender and puree until a smooth mixture is formed.
- Serve chilled after adding the crushed almonds.

Tip: A good resource for restoring Muscle Glycogen.

Banana Delight (Pre-Run)

A smoothie rich in low GI carbohydrates ideal when drunk pre-run. It provides a boost to the energy levels of the runner over longer periods of time and as such is great for long distance running. Bananas help in relaxing the gastrointestinal tract and do not upset the digestive system.

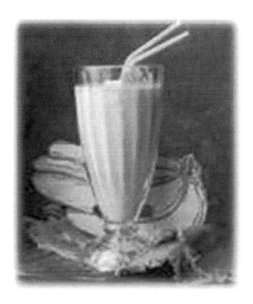

Preparation time	10 minutes
Ready time	10 minutes
Calories	467 cal
Total Fat	6.2 g
Cholesterol	24 mg
Sodium	231 mg
Total Carbohydrates	82.6 g
Dietary fibers	6.1 g
Sugars	58 g
Protein	20.6 g
Vitamin C	0.38
Vitamin A	0.1
Iron	0.05
Calcium	0.61

Ingredients

- 2 bananas
- 1 cup low-fat yoghurt
- ½ cup milk(skimmed)
- 1 teaspoon honey
- 1 cup ice

Method

- Mix all the ingredients in a blender and puree until a smooth mixture is formed.
- Serve with ice.

Tip: Bananas, low-fat yoghurt and skimmed milk are good sources of carbohydrates, fiber and protein.

Dates Boost (Pre-Run)

This smoothie gives the runner stamina to run fast and for long distances. Dates a natural resource for energy and as usual banana relaxes the gastrointestinal tract. As an added extra, protein powder can be added to make the smoothie more nutritious still.

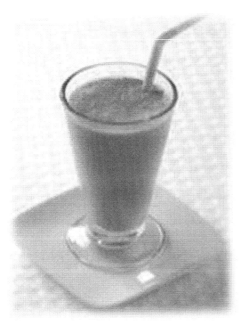

Preparation time	10 minutes
Ready time	10 minutes
Calories	617 Cal
Total Fat	19.5 g
Cholesterol	12 mg
Sodium	110 mg
Total Carbohydrates	107.2 g
Dietary fibers	10.9 g
Sugars	83.7 g
Protein	12.7 g
Vitamin C	0.18
Vitamin A	0.11
Iron	0.08
Calcium	0.35

Ingredients

- 1 banana
- ½ cup pitted dates
- 4 almonds
- 1tablespoon flaxseed oil
- 1 cup low-fat milk
- Pinch of cinnamon

Method

- Mix all the ingredients in a blender and puree until a smooth mixture is formed.
- Serve with ice and mint leaves.

Tip: Protein powder can be added to give this smoothie a boost.

Cocoa Smoothie (Pre-Run)

A low GI Carbohydrate smoothie is the best smoothie to help a runner to store enough glycogen which helps in running and maintains the glucose level for a longer time.

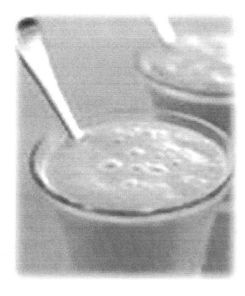

Preparation time	5 minutes
Ready time	5 minutes
Calories	229 Cal
Total Fat	4.0 g
Cholesterol	12 mg
Sodium	111mg
Total Carbohydrates	45.5 g
Dietary fibers	7.6 g
Sugars	32.2 g
Protein	10.8 g
Vitamin C	0.1
Vitamin A	0.1
Iron	0.11
Calcium	0.32

Ingredients

- 3 tablespoon cocoa powder
- 1 pear (chopped)
- 2 cup low-fat milk
- 2 teaspoon honey
- Pinch of cardamom

Method

- Mix all the ingredients in a blender except cardamom and mix until a smooth mixture is formed.
- Sprinkle with cardamom and serve chilled.

Tip: A low GI carbohydrate diet is the best Pre-Run smoothie to give energy enough to resist the strains of running.

Frisky Smoothie (Post-Run)

This smoothie is rich in high GI carbohydrates which should be had after the race in order to restore the sugar levels in the body. Almonds are rich in proteins which help to rejuvenate the muscles.

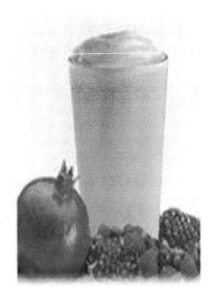

Preparation time	5 minutes
Ready time	5 minutes
Calories	266 Cal
Total Fat	4.2g
Cholesterol	4mg
Sodium	65mg
Total Carbohydrates	52.9 g
Dietary fibers	2.3 g
Sugars	40.7 g
Protein	5.7 g
Vitamin C	0.09
Vitamin A	0.05
Iron	0.02
Calcium	0.16

Ingredients

- 2 cups pomegranate juice
- 1 banana
- 10 almonds
- 1 cup low fat flavored milk

Method

- Mix all the ingredients in a blender and mix until a smooth mixture is formed.
- Add ice and drink chilled.

Tip: The almonds are good source of proteins which help in the wear and tear of tissue after running.

Banana Delight Smoothie (Post-Run)

Bananas replenish the potassium content lost due to excessive sweating. They reduce cramping caused by running and are a rich source of carbohydrates.

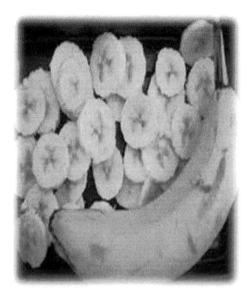

Preparation time	10 minutes
Ready time	10 minutes
Calories	277 Cal
Total Fat	2.7 G
Cholesterol	6 mg
Sodium	79 mg
Total Carbohydrates	59.3 g
Dietary fibers	3.2 g
Sugars	46.0 g
Protein	7.9 g
Vitamin C	1.03
Vitamin A	0.06
Iron	0.05
Calcium	0.16

Ingredients

- 2 bananas
- 1 cup apple juice
- 1 cup low-fat milk
- 1 cup low fat yoghurt
- 1 tablespoon honey

Method

- Mix all the ingredients in a blender and puree until a smooth mixture is formed.
- Serve chilled.

Tip: Bananas are a good source of carbohydrates essential for runners.

Fruitilicious Smoothie (Post-Run)

This smoothie has a combination of fruits which are rich in sugars hence they help to energize the body after a long run.

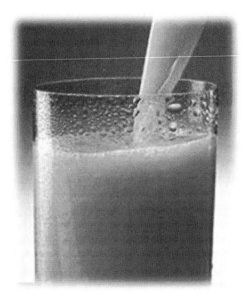

Preparation time	10 minutes
Ready time	10 minutes
Calories	340 Cal
Total Fat	15.0G
Cholesterol	0mg
Sodium	12 mg
Total Carbohydrates	55.4 g
Dietary fibers	8.0g
Sugars	40.8g
Protein	3.8g
Vitamin C	2.02
Vitamin A	0.22
Iron	0.09
Calcium	0.07

Ingredients

- 1 pineapple
- 1 mango
- ½ cup coconut milk
- 1 banana
- 1 orange

Method

- Mix all the ingredients in a blender and puree until a smooth mixture is formed.
- Serve with ice and sprinkle with cinnamon powder.

Tip: Fruits are the best source of vitamins which are required in higher quantities by runners.

Chocolate Smoothie (Post-Run)

This smoothie is a creamy one with high GI carbohydrates which help to restore the wear and tear of the tissues and restores the energy levels too.

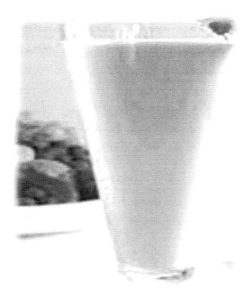

Preparation time	10 minutes
Ready time	10 minutes
Calories	96 Cal
Total Fat	3.2 G
Cholesterol	10mg
Sodium	51mg
Total Carbohydrates	14.7 g
Dietary fibers	2.3g
Sugars	11.2 g
Protein	5.1g
Vitamin C	0.03
Vitamin A	0.05
Iron	0.05
Calcium	0.15

Ingredients

- 1 cup milk(low fat)
- 2 tablespoons cocoa powder
- ½ cup chopped apple
- Pinch of cardamom
- 1 teaspoon sugar

Method

- Mix all the ingredients in a blender and puree until a smooth mixture is formed.
- Serve with ice and sprinkle with cardamom powder.

Tip: This smoothie has high GI carbohydrates.

Chocó- Coffee Smoothie (Pre-Run)

This chocolate recipe has high GI carbohydrates which provide energy for restoring the body to its previous state after a heavy workout or race.

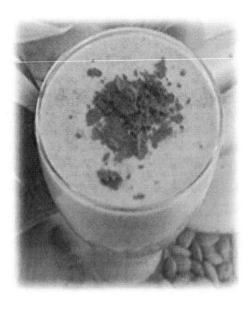

Preparation time	10 minutes
Ready time	10 minutes
Calories	167 Cal
Total Fat	5.2 G
Cholesterol	14mg
Sodium	98mg
Total Carbohydrates	23.1 g
Dietary fibers	0.5g
Sugars	20.9 g
Protein	7.2g
Vitamin C	0.01
Vitamin A	0.06
Iron	0.02
Calcium	0.16

Ingredients

- 1 cup low fat yoghurt
- 1 cup milk
- 1 teaspoon coffee powder
- 1 teaspoon chocolate powder
- 4 tablespoon Cream
- 2 teaspoon sugar

Method

- Mix all the ingredients in a blender and puree until a smooth mixture is formed.
- Add ice and sprinkle with chocolate powder.

Tip: High in calcium content with high GI carbohydrates due to the cream's caloric value.

Mango Smoothie (Post-Run)

Mango is rich source of sugar and hence is good for replenishing energy for runners. This smoothie is high in GI carbohydrate which is recommended for runners to restore the glycogen content in the body.

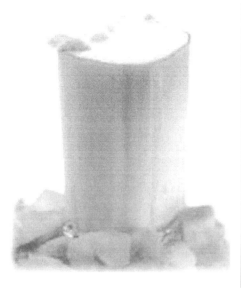

Preparation time	10 minutes
Ready time	10 minutes
Calories	408 Cal
Total Fat	6.9 g
Cholesterol	27 mg
Sodium	191 mg
Total Carbohydrates	72.6 g
Dietary fibers	3.8 g
Sugars	68.9 g
Protein	16.2 g
Vitamin C	0.98
Vitamin A	0.42
Iron	0.03
Calcium	0.53

Ingredients

- 2 ripe mango(pitted and chopped)
- 2 cups milk(low-fat)
- 2 tablespoons honey
- 1 cup low-fat yoghurt
- Pinch of cardamom powder

Method

- Mix all the ingredients in a blender and puree until a smooth mixture is formed.
- Serve with ice and sprinkle with cardamom powder.

Tip: This smoothie is high in GI carbohydrate which is recommended for runners to restore the glycogen content in the body

Fruity Punch (Post-Run)

The calcium provided by milk is needed for the wear and tear of bones and muscles too. Moreover the high sugar content makes it a high GI carbohydrate smoothie effective after a workout.

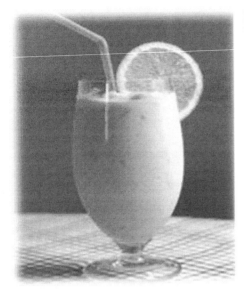

Preparation time	10 minutes
Ready time	10 minutes
Calories	287 Cal
Total Fat	5.3 g
Cholesterol	20 mg
Sodium	102 mg
Total Carbohydrates	54.3 g
Dietary fibers	4.2 g
Sugars	40.2 g
Protein	9.8 g
Vitamin C	0.8
Vitamin A	0.12
Iron	0.04
Calcium	0.3

Ingredients

- 1 cup pineapple(chopped)
- 2 cups milk(skimmed)
- 2 bananas
- 2 teaspoons honey

Method

- Mix all the ingredients in a blender and puree until a smooth mixture is formed.
- Serve with ice.

Tip: Banana and Pineapple, both are rich in Vitamin C which helps to restore glycogen in the body.

Butter milk Smoothies (Pre-Run)

Buttermilk is a tasty alternative to regular milk that's packed with carbohydrates and calcium. It is good to have as a pre-run snack as it will not disturb the GI tract.

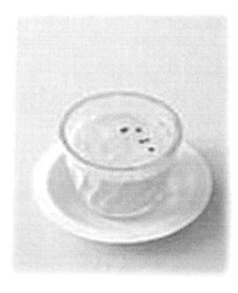

Preparation time	10 minutes
Ready time	10 minutes
Calories	312 Cal
Total Fat	1.4 g
Cholesterol	5 mg
Sodium	134 mg
Total Carbohydrates	70.9 g
Dietary fibers	0.5 g
Sugars	57.7 g
Protein	5.7 g
Vitamin C	0.59
Vitamin A	0.01
Iron	0.08
Calcium	0.23

Ingredients

- 2 cups fresh pineapple juice
- 1 cup buttermilk
- 2 cups pineapple sliced and crushed to small pieces
- 1 teaspoon honey

Method

- Mix all the ingredients in a blender and puree until a smooth mixture is formed.
- Serve with ice.

Tip: Buttermilk is good replacement for milk and yoghurt. It gives a high carbohydrate content and calcium too.

Oats Smoothie (Pre-Run)

This smoothie takes care for the runners pre-run requirements and is the best diet supplement for marathon runners or runners who are going for a heavy workout. Oats are the best carbohydrate source in the morning and are added in this smoothie too.

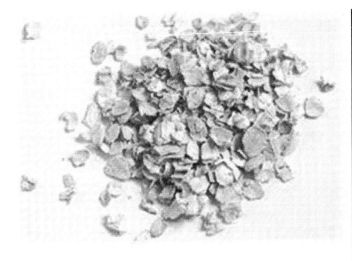

Preparation time	10 minutes
Ready time	10 minutes
Calories	300 Cal
Total Fat	6.1 g
Cholesterol	12 mg
Sodium	130 mg
Total Carbohydrates	45.7 g
Dietary fibers	4.8 g
Sugars	18 g
Protein	16.2 g
Vitamin C	0.35
Vitamin A	0.1
Iron	0.11
Calcium	0.32

Ingredients

- 1 cup Quaker oats
- 2 cups of low-fat milk
- ½ cup low fat yoghurt
- ½ cup strawberries chopped

Method

- Here it is required to heat the oats with milk to prepare like porridge.
- The ingredients in blend all the ingredients in a blender and puree until a smooth mixture is formed.
- Drink chilled.
- This smoothie is rich in oats which are recommended as an energy booster before a long run or workout.

Pineapple Coconut Smoothie (Post-Run)

This recipe is rich in GI carbohydrate which makes it great for replenishing energy after a heavy workout or after running for a long distance.

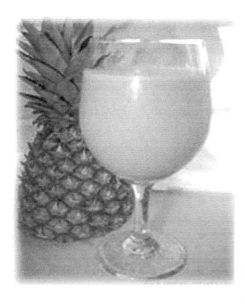

Preparation time	10 minutes
Ready time	10 minutes
Calories	239 Cal
Total Fat	14.5 g
Cholesterol	0 mg
Sodium	14 mg
Total Carbohydrates	29.3 g
Dietary fibers	3.7 g
Sugars	20.7 g
Protein	2.4 g
Vitamin C	1.01
Vitamin A	0.02
Iron	0.08
Calcium	0.03

Ingredients

- ½ pineapple sliced
- 1 banana
- 1 cup Coconut milk
- ½ cup strawberry juice

Method

- Mix all the ingredients in a blender and puree until a smooth mixture is formed.
- Drink chilled.

Tip: A high GI carbohydrate diet is the best Post-Run smoothie to rejuvenate the body.

Power- Packed Smoothie (Post-Run)

This smoothie has a combination of fruits and is a high GI carbohydrates drink. It is the best recipe for post-workout drinks. It recovers the body fast and gives a boost to the stamina after a long run. The Flaxseeds are a great source of nutrition for athletes. Aloe Vera in this recipe is a diuretic which helps to keep the body functioning smoothly.

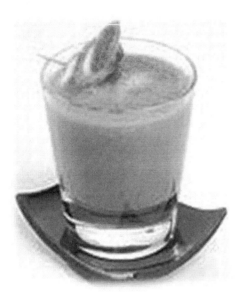

Preparation time	5 minutes
Ready time	5 minutes
Serves	1
Serving quantity/unit	510 G / 18 Ounces
Calories	310 Cal
Total Fat	4g
Cholesterol	0mg
Sodium	36mg
Total Carbohydrates	68g
Dietary fibers	19 g
Sugars	41 g
Protein	11g

Ingredients

- 3 bananas
- ½ tablespoon aloe Vera
- 1 cup almond milk
- 1 cup of chopped papaya
- ½ teaspoon flax seeds

Method

- Mix all the ingredients in a blender and puree until a smooth mixture is formed.
- Drink chilled.

Tip: This smoothie has flax seeds which is very good food for helping athletes to maintain their energy levels.

Multivitamin Smoothies

Vitamins are essential for Runners in order to maintain a healthy body. Multivitamins not only provide good health but also help in to gain endurance and support peak performance. The best way to get multivitamins is through natural sources. Medical experts often advise athletes who are always exercising and toning their bodies to ensure a higher intake of multivitamins. Runners require a higher level of endurance which multivitamins can help achieve. Athletes need more vitamins as they burn more calories and often need a lot of energy to meet the challenges of their chosen sport.

A high dose of multivitamins can be had by mixing various natural ingredients which provide vitamins. Smoothies are blended fruits or vegetables along with other ingredients and these provide a high dose of vitamins instantly to support the daily requirements of athletes.

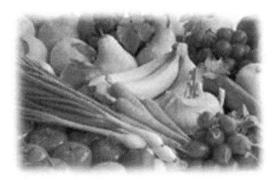

Blueberry-Avocado Punch (Pre-Run)

This smoothie contains blueberries and avocado which are rich in vitamins and minerals like potassium and zinc and many others. This power-packed smoothie keeps you energized for a long time.

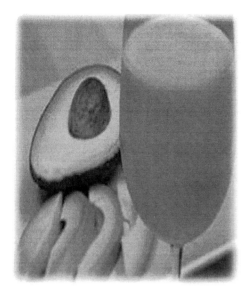

Preparation time	5 minutes
Ready time	5 minutes
Serves	1
Serving quantity/unit	510 G / 18 Ounces
Calories	310 Cal
Total Fat	4g
Cholesterol	0mg
Sodium	36mg
Total Carbohydrates	68g
Dietary fibers	19 g
Sugars	41 g
Protein	11g

Ingredients

- 1 cup blueberries
- 2 bananas
- 1 tablespoon avocado
- 1 lettuce chopped
- 1 cup water

Method

- Take all the ingredients except the lettuce and mix all the ingredients in a blender.
- Add the lettuce and puree until a smooth mixture is formed.
- Serve with ice and mint leaves.

Tip: This smoothie is rich in potassium and zinc which is energizing.

Vegetable Smoothie (Post-Run)

Vegetables are essential for runners as they are natural resources of proteins and fiber. Moreover they are a rich source of vitamins essential for the functioning of the body. Broccoli is good to keep the cardio-vascular muscles in check.

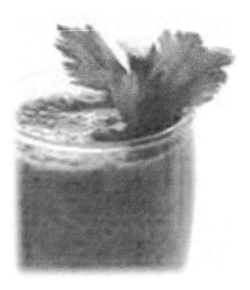

Preparation time	5 minutes
Ready time	5 minutes
Serves	1
Serving quantity/unit	510 G / 18 Ounces
Calories	310 Cal
Total Fat	4g
Cholesterol	0mg
Sodium	36mg
Total Carbohydrates	68g
Dietary fibers	19 g
Sugars	41 g
Protein	11g

Ingredients

- 1 banana
- 2 cups of spinach chopped
- 1 apple diced
- 1 cup chopped broccoli
- 3 tablespoons yoghurt

Method

- Mix all the ingredients in a blender along with a cup of water and puree until a smooth mixture is formed.
- Serve with ice.

Tip: Green vegetables are the best source of minerals essential for the pre-run breakfast.

Smoothies Rich in Vitamin C (Post-Run)

Running often causes wearing of tissues. Vitamin C is very essential for minimizing and recovering from wear and tear of the tissues in the body. They help in the maintenance of cartilages, bones and the teeth also. Hence this Vitamin C rich smoothie is good for supporting the increased nutritional requirements of athletes and can be had any time of the day.

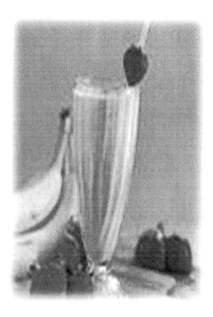

Preparation time	5 minutes
Ready time	5 minutes
Serves	1
Serving quantity/unit	510 G / 18 Ounces
Calories	310 Cal
Total Fat	4g
Cholesterol	0mg
Sodium	36mg
Total Carbohydrates	68g
Dietary fibers	19 g
Sugars	41 g
Protein	11g

Ingredients

- 1 banana
- 4 tablespoon of orange juice
- ½ cup chopped strawberries
- 1/4th cup chopped peaches
- 1 teaspoon honey

Method

- Mix all the ingredients in a blender and puree until a smooth mixture is formed.
- Serve with ice and mint leaves.

Tip: Bananas are unlikely to affect the GI tract and are a very good source of carbohydrates hence this smoothie can be had before running too.

Cherries Smoothie (Pre-Run)

The cherries provide vitamins whereas the low fat yoghurt is rich in carbohydrates and proteins and also calcium too. Calcium is good for the bones and reduces the chance of developing stress fractures.

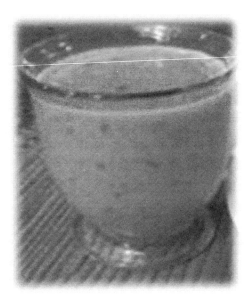

Preparation time	5 minutes
Ready time	5 minutes
Serves	1
Serving quantity/unit	510 G / 18 Ounces
Calories	310 Cal
Total Fat	4g
Cholesterol	0mg
Sodium	36mg
Total Carbohydrates	68g
Dietary fibers	19 g
Sugars	41 g
Protein	11g

Ingredients

- 2 cups cherries(finely chopped)
- 1 cup soy-milk (flavored)
- 1 cup low-fat yoghurt
- 1 teaspoon honey

Method

- Mix all the ingredients in a blender and puree until a smooth mixture is formed.
- Drink chilled...

Tip: The cherries are rich in vitamins and calcium is provided by other ingredients.

Rehydrating Smoothies (Post-Run)

The best way to rejuvenate after a long run is by rehydration. Water is the best rehydrating agent. Watermelon is a good rehydrating agent and so is coconut water. Drink this to rehydrate quickly after an intense workout.

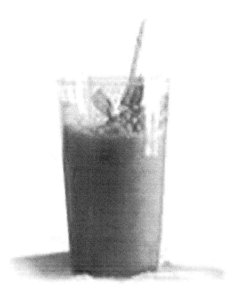

Preparation time	5 minutes
Ready time	5 minutes
Serves	1
Serving quantity/unit	510 G / 18 Ounces
Calories	310 Cal
Total Fat	4g
Cholesterol	0mg
Sodium	36mg
Total Carbohydrates	68g
Dietary fibers	19 g
Sugars	41 g
Protein	11g

Ingredients

- 1 cup coconut juice
- 2 cups of watermelon juice
- Vanilla flavored cream
- Ice cubes

Method

- Mix all the ingredients in a blender and puree until a smooth mixture is formed.
- Serve with ice.

Tip: Rehydration is required after a long run and is provided by coconut water and watermelon juice.

Vitamin A Rich Smoothie (Pre-Run)

Carrots are a rich source of Vitamin A and are not filling yet they are rich in calories. This makes the smoothie an excellent choice for before running as an energy booster.

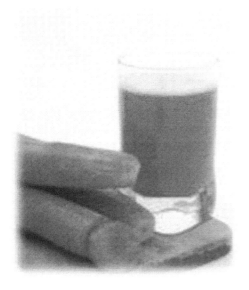

Preparation time	5 minutes
Ready time	5 minutes
Serves	1
Serving quantity/unit	510 G / 18 Ounces
Calories	310 Cal
Total Fat	4g
Cholesterol	0mg
Sodium	36mg
Total Carbohydrates	68g
Dietary fibers	19 g
Sugars	41 g
Protein	11g

Ingredients

- 1 cup carrots(finely chopped)
- 1 cup orange juice
- 1 teaspoon orange peel
- 1 teaspoon honey

Method

- Mix all the ingredients in a blender and puree until a smooth mixture is formed.
- Drink chilled.

Tip: This smoothie is rich in Vitamin A and it is essential for increasing the immunity. This recipe is quite filling yet low in calories.

Carrot Smoothie (Pre-Run)

This smoothie has carrots which are appropriate for promoting immunity owing to the presence of Vitamin A. This smoothie is rich in fiber content and sugars which make it an ideal pre run smoothie.

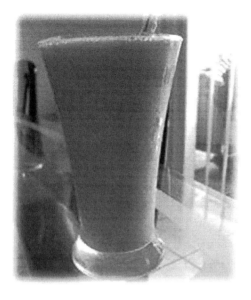

Preparation time	5 minutes
Ready time	5 minutes
Serves	1
Serving quantity/unit	510 G / 18 Ounces
Calories	310 Cal
Total Fat	4g
Cholesterol	0mg
Sodium	36mg
Total Carbohydrates	68g
Dietary fibers	19 g
Sugars	41 g
Protein	11g

Ingredients

- 2 carrots
- 2 apricots
- 2 cups spinach
- 1 cup water
- 1 tablespoon honey

Method

- Mix all the ingredients in a blender and puree until a smooth mixture is formed.
- Serve with ice.

Tip: This smoothie is rich in iron and vitamins.

Carrot Tomato Delight (Post-Run)

The vitamins C and A are helpful in restoring the immunity and also help in rejuvenating the body after a long run or workout.

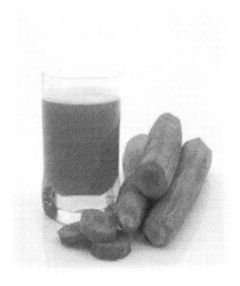

Preparation time	5 minutes
Ready time	5 minutes
Serves	1
Serving quantity/unit	510 G / 18 Ounces
Calories	310 Cal
Total Fat	4g
Cholesterol	0mg
Sodium	36mg
Total Carbohydrates	68g
Dietary fibers	19 g
Sugars	41 g
Protein	11g

Ingredients

- 2 carrots grated
- 3 tomatoes
- 2 tablespoon lemon juice
- ¼ cup chopped Celery
- Mint leaves
- Salt to taste

Method

- Mix all the ingredients in a blender and puree until a smooth mixture is formed.
- Serve with ice and mint leaves.

Tip: Carrots and tomatoes are rich sources of Vitamin A and Vitamin C respectively. A rejuvenating smoothie...

Kiwi Cooler (Pre-Run)

Green tea consists of antioxidant which is good for speedy recovery of injuries and also reduces the soreness. Kiwi is a rich source of Vitamin C which gives a boost to the wear and tear of the body.

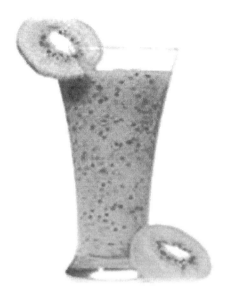

Preparation time	5 minutes
Ready time	5 minutes
Serves	1
Serving quantity/unit	510 G / 18 Ounces
Calories	310 Cal
Total Fat	4g
Cholesterol	0mg
Sodium	36mg
Total Carbohydrates	68g
Dietary fibers	19 g
Sugars	41 g
Protein	11g

Ingredients

- 1 kiwi chopped
- 1 cup pineapple chopped
- 2 teaspoon honey
- ½ cup green tea
- Ice cubes

Method

- Mix all the ingredients in a blender mix until a smooth mixture is formed.
- Add ice and drink.

Tip: A powerful anti oxidant which helps lessen the injuries pain and also helps reduce the chance of injury whilst also speeding recovery.

Protein Rich Smoothies

Proteins are essential to enable muscle growth. When incorporated in the smoothies along with carbohydrates they slow the digestion of carbohydrates.

Proteins also help in strengthening the immune system of the body and shielding the body against injury as the proteins helps to heal the body.

Proteins are also essential to ensure the effective functioning of the immune system. They increase the production of white blood cells which help the body to fight against diseases.

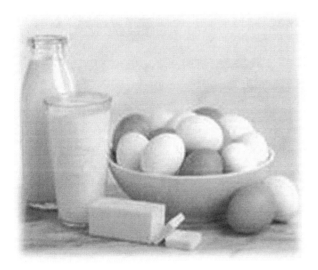

Chocolate Smoothie with Peanut Butter (Pre-Run)

Peanut butter is a rich source of protein and it helps make you feel full. This smoothie is rich in protein and fiber too. It is a wholesome food and this is a good smoothie before running if not overdone.

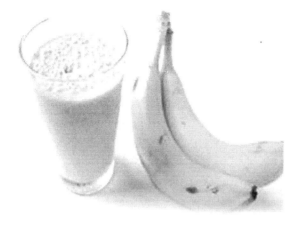

Preparation time	5 minutes
Ready time	5 minutes
Serves	1
Serving quantity/unit	510 G / 18 Ounces
Calories	310 Cal
Total Fat	4g
Cholesterol	0mg
Sodium	36mg
Total Carbohydrates	68g
Dietary fibers	19 g
Sugars	41 g
Protein	11g

Ingredients

- 1/2 cup chocolate-milk(low-fat)
- 2 cups milk(skimmed)
- 2 tablespoons peanut butter
- 3 bananas

Method

- Mix all the ingredients in a blender and puree until a smooth mixture is formed.
- Serve with ice and sprinkle with chocolate powder.

Tip: Peanut butter is a source of proteins which are necessary for repairing the muscles while doing workout.

Banana with Peanut Butter Smoothie (Pre-Run)

Peanut butter is rich in proteins and fiber which helps the runners. Moreover bananas and yoghurt are rich sources of carbohydrates.

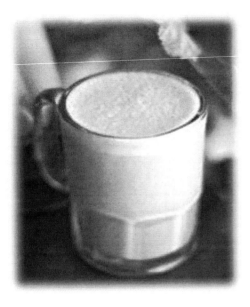

Preparation time	5 minutes
Ready time	5 minutes
Serves	1
Serving quantity/unit	510 G / 18 Ounces
Calories	310 Cal
Total Fat	4g
Cholesterol	0mg
Sodium	36mg
Total Carbohydrates	68g
Dietary fibers	19 g
Sugars	41 g
Protein	11g

Ingredients

- 2 teaspoons peanut butter
- 2 bananas
- 1 cup soy milk
- 1 cup low fat yoghurt
- 1 teaspoon honey

Method

- Mix all the ingredients in a blender and mix until a smooth mixture is formed.
- Add ice and drink chilled.

Tip: The peanut butter is good for runners as it is filling but does not make you fat.

Protein Smoothie (Post-Run)

This smoothie helps to recover from the wearing of tissues and really speeds up the recovery process after a long run. It reduces fatigue and is a great source of proteins too.

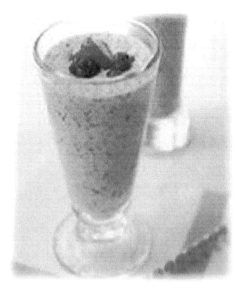

Preparation time	5 minutes
Ready time	5 minutes
Serves	1
Serving quantity/unit	510 G / 18 Ounces
Calories	310 Cal
Total Fat	4g
Cholesterol	0mg
Sodium	36mg
Total Carbohydrates	68g
Dietary fibers	19 g
Sugars	41 g
Protein	11g

Ingredients

- 1/2 cup blueberries
- 1 tablespoon Whey protein
- 1 cup low-fat milk
- ½ cup low fat yoghurt
- 1 banana

Method

- Mix all the ingredients in a blender and puree until a smooth mixture is formed.
- Serve with ice and sprinkle with chocolate powder.

Tip: The Whey protein is a natural rejuvenator for muscles.

Tofu Cherry Smoothie (Post-Run)

This smoothie is rich in beta-carotene due to the addition of tofu in it. It helps to rejuvenate the muscles and gives strength to the body.

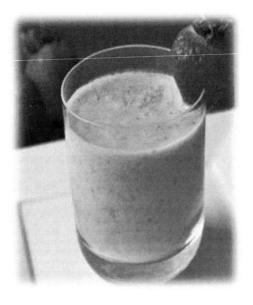

Preparation time	5 minutes
Ready time	5 minutes
Serves	1
Serving quantity/unit	510 G / 18 Ounces
Calories	310 Cal
Total Fat	4g
Cholesterol	0mg
Sodium	36mg
Total Carbohydrates	68g
Dietary fibers	19 g
Sugars	41 g
Protein	11g

Ingredients

- 1 cup soya milk
- 1 cup tofu
- 1 cup cherries
- 1 teaspoon honey

Method

- Mix all the ingredients in a blender and mix until a smooth mixture is formed.
- Add ice and drink chilled.

Tip: Make the smoothie just before drinking as tofu becomes dark if kept out for longer time.

Tofu Strawberry Smoothie (Post-Run)

This smoothie is rich in beta-carotene due to the addition of tofu in it. It helps to rejuvenate the muscles and gives strength to the body.

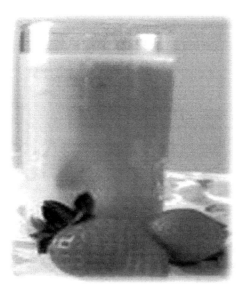

Preparation time	5 minutes
Ready time	5 minutes
Serves	1
Serving quantity/unit	510 G / 18 Ounces
Calories	310 Cal
Total Fat	4g
Cholesterol	0mg
Sodium	36mg
Total Carbohydrates	68g
Dietary fibers	19 g
Sugars	41 g
Protein	11g

Ingredients

- 3 cups strawberries (chopped)
- 4 tablespoons soft tofu
- 1 cup orange juice
- 2 teaspoon honey

Method

- Mix all the ingredients in a blender and mix until a smooth mixture is formed.
- Add ice and drink chilled.

Tip: The tofu is a great for helping to rejuvenate the muscles.

Eggs and Nutmeg Smoothie (Post-Run)

This smoothie is great for recovery due to its balance of protein and high GI carbohydrates.

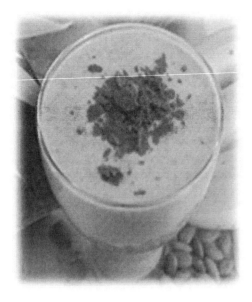

Preparation time	5 minutes
Ready time	5 minutes
Serves	1
Serving quantity/unit	510 G / 18 Ounces
Calories	310 Cal
Total Fat	4g
Cholesterol	0mg
Sodium	36mg
Total Carbohydrates	68g
Dietary fibers	19 g
Sugars	41 g
Protein	11g

Ingredients

- 1 banana
- 3 egg whites
- 1 cup low-fat milk
- 1 cup low fat yoghurt
- 1 tablespoon honey
- Nutmeg to sprinkle

Method

- Mix all the ingredients in a blender and puree until a smooth mixture is formed.
- Serve with ice and sprinkle with nutmeg powder.

Tip: The protein in the eggs rejuvenates the muscles. It is essential for the wear and tear of the muscles.

Protein Rich Pumpkin Smoothie (Post-Run)

This smoothie helps to recover the wearing of tissues and really speeds up the recovery process after a long run. It removes fatigue and is a great source of proteins too.

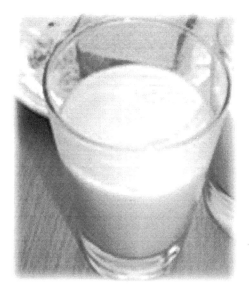

Preparation time	5 minutes
Ready time	5 minutes
Serves	1
Serving quantity/unit	510 G / 18 Ounces
Calories	310 Cal
Total Fat	4g
Cholesterol	0mg
Sodium	36mg
Total Carbohydrates	68g
Dietary fibers	19 g
Sugars	41 g
Protein	11g

Ingredients

- 1/2 cup milk(low fat)
- 1 cup yoghurt
- 1 cup chopped pumpkin
- Pinch of cinnamon
- 1 banana

Method

- Mix all the ingredients in a blender and puree until a smooth mixture is formed.
- Serve with ice and sprinkle with cinnamon powder.

Tip: Pumpkin is rich in Vitamin A.

Green Smoothies

Green smoothies are a very good source of carbohydrates and they are good for the blood sugar levels too. They contain high fiber content which is useful to reduce the intake of sugar. As the vegetables are consumed raw, they retain all of their natural goodness. They are made up of low GI carbohydrates and hence are extremely effective Pre Run Smoothies.

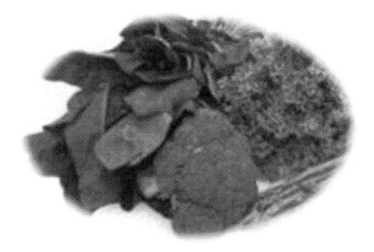

Pineapple Spinach Smoothie (Pre-Run)

The green vegetables have low GI carbohydrates and hence are suitable to drink before workouts and races. The green smoothies are good enough to take care of the sugar intake and also provide nutrition to the body.

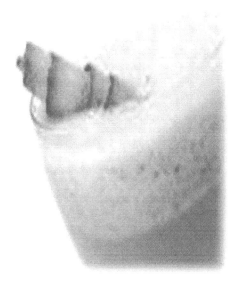

Preparation time	5 minutes
Ready time	5 minutes
Serves	1
Serving quantity/unit	510 G / 18 Ounces
Calories	310 Cal
Total Fat	4g
Cholesterol	0mg
Sodium	36mg
Total Carbohydrates	68g
Dietary fibers	19 g
Sugars	41 g
Protein	11g

Ingredients

- 2 cup pineapple(chopped)
- 2 cups spinach chopped
- 2 cups of pineapple juice
- ½ cup of yoghurt(low-fat)
- Dark chocolate chips

Method

- Mix all the ingredients in a blender and puree until a smooth mixture is formed.
- Serve with ice.

Tip: Spinach and Pineapple, both are rich in Vitamin C which helps to restore glycogen in the body.

Vitamins Rich Smoothie (Post-Run)

This smoothie helps to recover the wearing of tissues and really speeds up the recovery process after a long run. It removes fatigue and is a great source of proteins too.

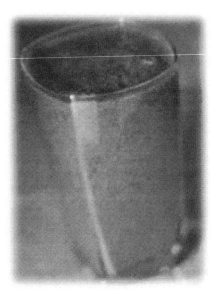

Preparation time	5 minutes
Ready time	5 minutes
Serves	1
Serving quantity/unit	510 G / 18 Ounces
Calories	310 Cal
Total Fat	4g
Cholesterol	0mg
Sodium	36mg
Total Carbohydrates	68g
Dietary fibers	19 g
Sugars	41 g
Protein	11g

Ingredients

- 1 apricot
- 1 cup orange juice
- 1 cup spinach
- Piece of ginger
- 2 bananas

Method

- Mix all the ingredients in a blender and puree until a smooth mixture is formed along with two cups of water.
- Serve with ice.

Tip: This is a high vitamins drink and makes the runner rejuvenated before any workout.

Cooler Smoothie (Pre-Run)

Peanut butter is rich in proteins and fiber which helps the runners. Moreover bananas and yoghurt are rich sources of carbohydrates.

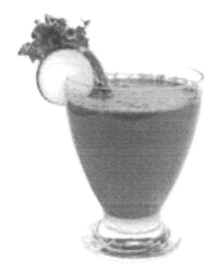

Preparation time	5 minutes
Ready time	5 minutes
Serves	1
Serving quantity/unit	510 G / 18 Ounces
Calories	310 Cal
Total Fat	4g
Cholesterol	0mg
Sodium	36mg
Total Carbohydrates	68g
Dietary fibers	19 g
Sugars	41 g
Protein	11g

Ingredients

- ½ cup cucumber
- 2 bananas
- 1 kiwi
- 1 cup spinach
- 2 cups water

Method

- Mix all the ingredients in a blender and mix until a smooth mixture is formed.
- Add ice and drink chilled.

Tip: The smoothie is good in summers as it has cucumber which provides a cooling effect to the body.

Spinach with Oats Smoothie (Pre-Run)

This smoothie takes care for the runners pre-run requirements and is the best diet supplement for marathon runners or runners who are going for a heavy workout. Oats are the best carbohydrate source in the morning and are added in this smoothie too. Spinach and Banana provide sugars and vitamins.

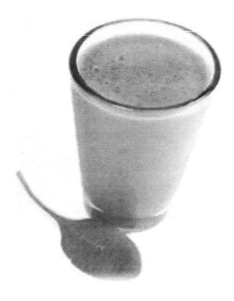

Preparation time	5 minutes
Ready time	5 minutes
Serves	1
Serving quantity/unit	510 G / 18 Ounces
Calories	310 Cal
Total Fat	4g
Cholesterol	0mg
Sodium	36mg
Total Carbohydrates	68g
Dietary fibers	19 g
Sugars	41 g
Protein	11g

Ingredients

- 1/2 cup Quaker oats
- 1 banana
- 1cup mango pieces
- 2 cups of spinach
- 1cup water

Method

- Here it is required to heat the oats with water for 2 minutes and cool.
- Then blend all the ingredients in a blender and puree until a smooth mixture is formed. Drink chilled.

Tip: This smoothie is rich in oats which are recommended as an energy booster before a long run or workout. Banana is good for energizing and also relaxes the GI tract.

Refresher Smoothie (Pre-Run)

This smoothie is rich in vitamins and it has honey which is essential for a splurge of energy for the runners. A refreshing smoothie that will energize the whole body.

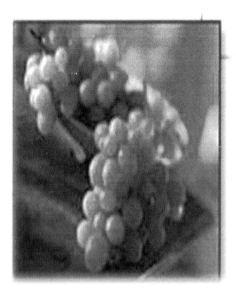

Preparation time	5 minutes
Ready time	5 minutes
Serves	1
Serving quantity/unit	510 G / 18 Ounces
Calories	310 Cal
Total Fat	4g
Cholesterol	0mg
Sodium	36mg
Total Carbohydrates	68g
Dietary fibers	19 g
Sugars	41 g
Protein	11g

Ingredients

- 1 cup green grapes
- 1 green apple
- 1cup apple juice
- 1 teaspoon honey

Method

- Mix all the ingredients in a blender and mix until a smooth mixture is formed.
- Add ice and drink chilled.

Tip: This smoothie is best enjoyed just before a run as it has low GI carbohydrates and provides sustained energy to the body.

Exclusive Bonus Download: Distance Running

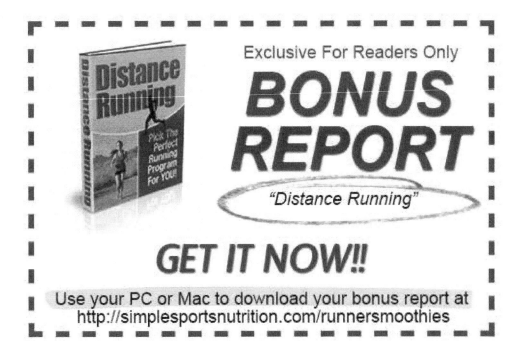

Download your bonus, please visit the download link above from your PC or MAC. To open PDF files, visit http://get.adobe.com/reader/ to download the reader if it's not already installed on your PC or Mac. To open ZIP files, you may need to download WinZip from http://www.winzip.com. This download is for PC or Mac ONLY and might not be downloadable to kindle.

Discover How You Can Increase Your Running In A Matter Of A Few Months!

Now, you can implement the same kind of training that runners use to train for marathons, races and other running events! You can steal the strategies that runners use to get to the next level. You will be able to discover the secrets that they use to get to where they are at today.

If your running speed is not up to par, this report, " Distance Running - Pick The Perfect Running Program For YOU! " , can help you get up to speed on the level that you need to be at with your running. There are six different running programs that explain how you can do just that, along with other tips that are crucial to your running success. This could be the most important thing that you will ever read to make those strides that you need to make in your running pursuits. This report will explain how you can train to be like some of the other runners that are involved in different races and marathons. Before you know it, you will be running in some of the most well-known running events and being able to win, just because of the training that you received.

You will learn about the training involved:

- One of the first thing that you have to do every day while you're training
- How to keep your back and hamstrings strong
- What kind of training to incorporate on the weekends
- The average distance that you should train
- Why you should have a schedule
- How many days a week runners train
- What you should incorporate in your training
- What you should do in between training and running
- And Much Much More!

Visit the URL above to download this guide and start achieving your weight loss and fitness goals NOW

One Last Thing...

Thank you so much for reading my book. I hope you really liked it. As you probably know, many people look at the reviews on Amazon before they decide to purchase a book. If you liked the book, could you please take a minute to leave a review with your feedback? 60 seconds is all I'm asking for, and it would mean the world to me.

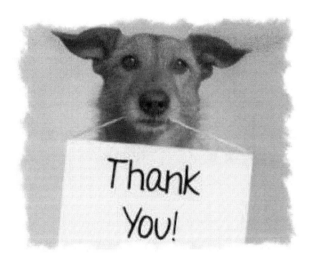

******

Books by This Author

The Smoothies for Runners Book

Juices for Runners

Smoothies for Cyclists

Juices for Cyclists

Paleo Diet for Cyclists

Smoothies for Triathletes

Juices for Triathletes

Paleo Diet for Triathletes

<u>Smoothies for Strength</u>

<u>Juices for Strength</u>

<u>Paleo Diet for Strength</u>

<u>Paleo Diet Smoothies for Strength</u>

<u>Smoothies for Golfers</u>

<u>Juices for Golfers</u>

About the Author

Lars Andersen is a sports author, nutritional researcher and fitness enthusiast. In his spare time he participates in competitive running, swimming and cycling events and enjoys hiking with his two border collies.

Lars Andersen

Published by Nordic Standard Publishing

Atlanta, Georgia USA

NORDICSTANDARD
PUBLISHING

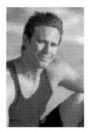

Copyright © 2012 Lars Andersen

Images and Cover by Nordic Standard Publishing

22513933R00029

Made in the USA
Lexington, KY
03 May 2013